Marketing Your Chair-Massage Business

Second Edition

A step-by-step, simple, effective guide to building a chair-massage practice

Technique instructions in this book and Youtube.com

I0449934

By Mark W. Worrell, L.C.M.T.

Table of Contents

Introduction   5

Part One: Attributes for Success   7
    Consistency   7
    Be Professional   8
    Commitment   10
    Conviction   10
    Confidence   11
    Be a Good Listener   12

Part Two: Acquiring Accounts   13
    Corporate Accounts   14
    "Front Door" Method   18
    Meeting your Contact Person   22
    "Back Door" Method   26
    Other Venues – different approaches   27
    "Fish Bowl" of Business   30
    Websites and Social Networking   31

Part Three: Maintaining your Accounts   35
    On Massage Day   35
    In-Office Promotional Flyer/Email   37
    Pricing   39
    Setting Goals   39
    Networking   40
    Promoting Full Body   41
    Now is the right time   42

Technique Instructions and Video on Youtube.com 43-53

Introduction

My name is Mark Worrell. I am a certified, licensed, and insured massage therapist. I have lived in the Los Angeles area all of my life. For the last 16 years, I have worked in massage, mainly earning my living through chair-massage accounts. The following pages outline the simplest and most effective marketing concepts that have helped me to acquire more than 25 accounts over the past 16 years.

I am writing this book to assist certified massage therapists in making a difference in this world and growing their chair-massage practices. This is a "no frills" kind of manual, so if you are looking for a lot of examples or stories on the life of a chair-massage therapist, this is probably not your "cup of tea." Through the years, I have lost accounts due to downsizing, relocating of companies, and the recent downturn in the economy. I regularly work in nine to 10 accounts a month. Usually, I visit a business every two to three weeks, and I work on five to 15 people a visit. I have taught chair-massage techniques and marketing for the past six years at various schools in the L.A. area and have instructed more than 250 students in chair massage. The basic chair massage lasts about 15 minutes. I do want to thank my students who encouraged me to write this all down and get this valuable information in book form. But remember, you have to do the work. I am just giving you a marketing plan so that you can find work yourself and become an entrepreneur.

Just like anything you learn, it's what you put into it that counts. Apply the effort and marketing tools in these pages and, just because it is a numbers game, you will eventually land your own chair-massage accounts. I believe that, over time, you can have a thriving chair-massage business. If you want, you could turn some of your chair-massage clients into regular full-body clients. It's up to you to get things done. This is a not a book that is getting business to "come to you" through just websites or a "pay per click" ad campaign. Physical paperwork designated to an individual person at a business is how you will get chair-massage accounts. This a book designed for you to go out and "get the business!"

My philosophy on massage therapy and competition is this: Do not worry about your colleagues. Every massage therapist in the world has a different touch from you as well as from me. I want to see massage therapy in every business and on every street corner, and chair massage is the best way to make that happen. In America, there's a little coffeehouse named Starbucks. Twenty-five years ago, it was just one shop in Seattle, Washington, and now it seems like they're on every other street corner. Now it's odd not to have one in your neighborhood. It is so commonplace that people expect it to be there. That's the way I feel about chair massage. I want it to be just as commonplace as Starbucks. I want every company in the U.S. to want this service for their employees. If that happened, I would not worry about competition, because there would be enough work for everyone.

Part One:
Attributes for Success

To start off, we will need to talk about some attributes that will help you personally with pursuing a successful chair-massage practice.

Of course, we all strive to be successful, but I really want to highlight these few attributes that stick out for me. Many students I have taught over the years express that getting motivated to just start marketing themselves is a daunting task. Clearly, the motivation for me has always been "putting food on the table." Literally! I have a mortgage, a car, two kids, a working spouse, and two cats to keep up. We have our IRAs set up for retirement. Plus, all the regular bills to keep up with.

But to say money is my main motivating factor would not be true. It's the lifestyle that I cherish and my relationships I have developed with my clients. I love being in a profession where people are happy to see me walk in the door. I work when I want to work, setting my own hours, charge a fair price for excellent service, and get to work on wonderful, health-minded individuals.

Consistency

Always follow through with phone calls, mailers, and making appointments. Be on time. Be reliable and flexible. Try to give the same massage every time.

The following pages ask you to make up "massage packages" to be mailed directly to businesses. Follow up with phone calls as well as making and keeping appointments. When I speak of giving the same massage every time, I mean it in the sense that you want to give the same service, always. Let's say that you were giving a deep-tissue stroke on the trapezius muscle, and your client especially liked that move. Your client booked you again the following week, but this time you skipped that deep-tissue stroke. She would not be too happy that you overlooked that stroke and probably would not book you again. I have consistently given the same basic chair-massage routine to the same clients over the last 12 years, and no one complains. They know what to expect and they get the same service every time. If a client walks in and says her neck is bothering her, of course I will spend the extra time working on her neck, but I always stick to the basic routine. When is the last time you had chocolate ice cream that tasted like strawberry? You ordered chocolate because you know what it tastes like.

Be Professional

In your appearance, in your personality, in your equipment—be certified, insured, and licensed.

If you are professionally trained as a massage therapist, you should always look the part. If you are going to a law firm,

8

slacks and a nice short-sleeve shirt are appropriate. If you go to a factory, jeans and a t-shirt are probably good enough. You have to know how to "read" the business that you are visiting. Creating respect for your profession is very important. If you dress in jeans and a t-shirt in a professional suit-and-tie business, they are not likely to invite you back because of your attire. That would be an unfortunate way to lose an account. If you are unsure, always dress "up," and after your first visit, you can make the determination on the appropriate outfit.

I happen to be a straight-forward, practical, talkative, and funny person. But I do consciously "tone down" my persona to fit my profession. Calm, gracious, and caring is my approach. I am there as a healer, not for entertainment or to "chat" it up. Knowing how your equipment works and how to make your client comfortable is very important. If your clients are not comfortable in any way, the likeliness that they book you again will diminish.

Certification and licensing can vary state to state or even city to city. It is up to you to determine where you are licensed and where you can practice legally. Insurance is important to have nowadays with the way people can get "sue happy" if you hurt them or if they have a reaction to your oils. Insurance should be the first thing you look into after you get certified. You can find applications in any massage magazine or search online. Typical massage insurance can cost as little as $100 per year. That should buy you approximately $3,000,000 worth of massage insurance.

Commitment

Commit to doing certain steps that are out of your "comfort zone" in order to create new opportunities.

The information that I present to you may not be something you feel comfortable attempting. It requires stepping out of your regular way of pursuing work in massage therapy. You are acting and speaking from the place of owning your own business through gaining massage accounts. It requires speaking to and meeting with people in positions of authority at a business. If you are used to going into a spa or chiropractic office and working for someone else who sets up your appointments with your clients, the following steps may challenge that "comfort zone." Get past it, be confident in yourself, and make it happen. You'll feel more confident each time you do the steps and follow through.

Conviction

Believe in what you are doing; your services are needed.

Realize that massage therapy is a necessity for many people. Receiving physical touch relieves stress, and many medical studies have proven that massage is indeed one of the best ways to relieve stress. Believe that your services are needed. The work will come.

Confidence

Know your massage therapy. Give as many free massages as necessary to feel comfortable in your application.

Research the best massage schools in your area that offer specific training in chair massage. Just because you have 500 hours in table work, doesn't mean you can automatically transfer that training to chair work. There is a definite difference in the application and approach. Try letting your friends or family members know that you need to practice a 15-minute chair-massage routine, and ask if you can work on them. "Great, I'd love to get a free chair massage," is usually the first response. Even though they may not be paying you for the massage, require that they give you **feedback** during the massage. No one told me this. Sixteen years ago, I would give a free massage and people would say, "Thanks—that was great!" I would respond with, "Well, what was the best part? Was the pressure ok? How did that stroke feel?" The problem was that I wasn't getting the feedback I needed at the actual moment of the massage to learn anything. So I suggest you ask every one to two minutes, "How's the pressure?" and "How does this feel?" Their payment to you is their honest opinion on the massage. You will learn much faster and become more confident with this information—and you can start to charge people sooner, knowing that you have a great massage routine. I tend to still ask people at least once during a regular chair massage if they are comfortable. Opening up a good line of communication with your clients will surely add to your service. They will feel more comfortable with you and feel that they are "heard."

Be a Good Listener

Listen to your clients' massage requests and their issues.

As you probably already have realized, in our profession, being a bodyworker, people tend to "open up" to you while receiving a massage. They talk about work, home life, the economy, and their family. When you first start working on them, you obviously want to respond to their comments and questions. But as time goes on during the massage, you also want to be less engaged in the conversation and just listen.

Another reason listening is important is you want to hear your clients' requests they might have for the massage. If they need more time spent on their arms and hands, make sure you do spend more of your time there. Receiving chair and full-body massages over the years, I have experienced a lot of therapists who have ignored or forgotten requests for extra attention during my massage sessions. Needless to say, I didn't book with them again.

Taking care of people requires listening skills and tender loving care. Remember, you won't have many return clients if they don't feel heard.

Part Two: Acquiring Accounts

When I speak of acquiring accounts, I mean that you are going to approach companies about giving chair massage to their employees on a regular basis (once a week, once a month, etc.)

Where do you want to work? Whom do you want to work on? I personally have no problem walking into any business and feeling comfortable. If you don't like lawyers, don't approach a law firm. I want to work on whoever wants to sit in my massage chair. With this approach I don't limit my clientele.

Suggestions:

- Offices: Law firms, insurance agencies, entertainment agencies, brokerage houses, marketing firms, movie studios, record companies, medical offices… any business with human bodies who are working!!

- Flea markets, grocery stores, health-food stores, shopping malls, and hair salons.

- Trade shows, conventions, and exhibits.

Corporate Accounts

Putting Together Your Massage Package

Cover letter

Start out your cover letter with the date at the top of the page, (skip a line), the company's name, contact name (you'll find out how to get this information in the following pages), and business address.

1. *Introduce yourself and chair massage.* Use your own style to introduce yourself, but in general you want to say, "Dear _____, my name is_____, and I am a certified, licensed, and insured massage therapist. I wanted to speak with you about offering chair massage to your employees."

2. *If you have worked in the area (geographically), mention the name of the account or person.* If you have performed any type of massage, e.g., at a massage school or a private client, go ahead and state it. Mention an account even if it is within 25 miles of their location. Find out what kind of business, e.g., law firm, insurance agency etc., and mention their stressors. If you were to mention catchwords like "depositions" or "litigations" to people at a law firm, they will understand that you're aware of what they do on a daily basis. You just want them to know that you are a "local" and you know about the stress that is involved with their business.

3. *Mention benefits of chair massage.* Reduces stress, calms the nervous system, boosts alertness. You can list these benefits in paragraph form or in bullet points. As a therapist, you obviously know the benefits. The more they know, the more they will realize that they need your services.

4. *Point out that massage improves employee morale.* By offering chair massage to its employees, a company is saying that it cares and wants to provide a pleasant work environment. A happy employee is a loyal employee! When it's massage day at an account, the employees are looking forward to the day and they are visibly happier.

5. *Mention the health and well-being of employees.* A lot of companies don't think about this one, but you are there to remind them. If they take care of their employees, their employees will take care of their business. Healthy employees are more productive and take off less sick days. Most accounts promote a "wellness program" that you can be the center of. Employees' stress levels at work are on the rise, but just by offering chair massage as part of a wellness program, those stress levels can be lowered.

6. *Cost can be paid by employees or shared with the employer.* Mention how long each massage is and what your rate is. Cost can be paid by the employee or, sometimes, shared with the employer. If they are interested enough, they might pick up the whole tab. But for now, you just want to get your foot in the door. When it comes time for a meeting, you can talk cost-sharing then.

7. *In-Closing*. Mention that you would like to meet to give them a *free* chair massage and talk about how this would be a wonderful idea for the company's employees. Say that you will be in touch in the next week or two. End with, "Sincerely, [your name and contact information]."

Resume

Contains education, training, where you currently offer massage, and past employment even if not massage related.

You need to tailor a massage resume with all of your educational background. Every massage course or workshop is relevant. If you are working at a spa or chiropractic office, definitely add that to your resume with dates of employment. Therapists differ when it comes to mentioning other careers they have had in the past that are not massage related. I personally believe that it is a good idea to mention every place that you have worked at, because it can show a history of maintaining a regular job.

Business cards

Contain name, title, phone number, and maybe a design.

Simpler is better. My belief is that you should not put too much information on a business card. Having every modality from shiatsu to deep tissue is too much for the average person to absorb. They might even feel intimidated or ignorant if they don't know what shiatsu is, and it might prevent them from calling. If you just have "Mark Worrell, Massage Therapist," they will understand what you do. If they know enough to want shiatsu, they will call to inquire. You just want to get them calling you, that's the point. When a business card is too busy, some studies have shown that it actually stresses people out. And that defeats the purpose of them contacting you.

Brochures

Chair-massage brochures give the client a visual of what chair massage is like.

You can make up your own brochure and personalize it if you like. The benefits of massage and your resume in paragraph form, pictures, and references are what make a good brochure. However, that is a lot of extra work. I particularly like to order pre-printed brochures that you can order from any massage magazine. You can even have your name and contact information printed on the back for an extra small fee. Go online to find other resources on massage brochures.

This is your "massage package". Now you have all this information together in a nice presentable form. The aim is to get all this information to the right individual at a company. Here's where it gets to be fun!

"Front Door" Method

A. *Target location of potential business to approach.*

(Example: Any office that has human bodies!) Target your location by driving to a business district or business center in your city. Park and get out with a notebook and pen handy. Walk the street for a few blocks and write down the names of businesses in each building you walk by. Enter any building lobby and walk up to the directory to write down the names of the businesses. Go home!

B. *Call information "411" or, better yet, get on the Internet.*

Search for business name, address, and phone number. Your main objective is to get the phone number.

C. *Call business and ask the receptionist: "Hi, can I get the name of your human resources manager or office manager, please?"*

Get the name, say thank you, and hang up the phone. Now, sometimes you will get a receptionist who is a little more inquisitive and might ask, *"What is this concerning?"* Best answer is that you would like to send them some information on employee benefits. At that point, the receptionist will probably give you the name because you sound like you know what you're talking about.

D. *Mail cover letter, resume, business card, and brochure in a nice off-white or earth-toned* *envelope with the contact person's name on the cover letter.*

Make sure you address the envelope with "ATTN: [Contact person's name] (e.g., Holly Brown)."

E. *Wait five to seven business days before calling and asking for the contact person.*

The reason for waiting this long is to give them time to receive and consider your proposal. I suggest calling between Tuesday and Thursday in the late morning hours. They will have gotten through the "rush" of the morning and be looking forward to lunchtime. Waiting those five to seven days will give them a chance to run it by someone in management who might be the decision maker in taking on your services. Your phone call is your first contact with the person and company, so rehearse a little with someone to get down your opening. I usually say, *"Hi Holly! My name is Mark Worrell. I am the certified massage therapist who sent you the information on chair massage last week. How are you?"* They usually answer, *"Fine, and how are you?"* I reply, *"I'm fantastic. I was hoping that sometime next week, I could pop in to give you a free chair massage so you can see firsthand how wonderful it is!"* Yes, ask for a meeting right away! You'll know instantly if they are interested. Instead of wasting time talking about how great chair massage would be for the company, ask for 20 minutes of their time. If the answer is yes, figure out a date and time that works for your schedules.

I'm not going to lie and say that you get a positive response every time. This is a numbers game, remember. If the person is not interested, ask politely if she will hold on to your information in case she reconsiders. Or, make sure to mention that you are available for any health fairs or employee appreciation days. Also, if time permits, again offer the free chair massage anytime in the near future. It all depends on how personable she is over the phone. You'll have to judge that call by call.

Keep a good record of businesses you've sent information to. The easiest way to do this is on 3x5 index cards... Yes, index cards. Call me old-fashioned, but the easiest way to forget the information you gather is to depend on a computer or mobile device. If you physically write down the information on the index cards, you will remember it better. Having the information in your cell phone or laptop can actually be inconvenient. Not to mention how they are more apt to be lost or stolen if you carry them around all the time. Having the business name, contact person, address, phone number, date mailed, and date of first phone call on a 3x5 index card is much more efficient. Having the cards with you when you make the calls allows you to take intricate notes on the conversation and whether or not they're interested or if "right now" is not the right time for your services. If that is the case, ask if you can call back in six months to say "hi."

Also, more than 90 percent of the time, you will get their voicemail. Be sure to leave all your contact information and ask for that meeting. Mention the free massage and that you only need 20 minutes of their time. Hopefully, they will call back in a day or two.

However, more than likely, you will have to call them a second time the following week. When you call the second time, write that date down on your index card. This so you don't call too often (scaring them away) or not often enough to keep you on their radar. If you get the voicemail again on the second call, leave the same information you left on the first call, but add that you will "be in their area next week for another meeting" and you'd love to "pop in" to give them a quick chair massage.

The idea here is to give them the impression that a) you have other interested companies that are looking for your services, and b) that you are quite flexible for a meeting that same day. Again, you are trying to entice them into a meeting and how easy it would be for them.

Meeting your Contact Person

1. Show up on time (early) with a fresh resume, business and personal references, brochure, and sign-up sheet. Sign-up sheets are really basic. You want your name, title, phone number, "SIGN UP SHEET", date of massage, massage times, and place for client's name and extension number in the office. Here's generally what it should look like:

Mark Worrell
Certified Massage Therapist
[Your phone number]

Date: Thurs. 8/13/09

Chair-massage sign-up sheet

Time	Name	Ext.#
11:00		
11:20		
11:40		
12:00		
12:20		
	LUNCH	
1:20		
1:40		
2:00		
2:20		
2:40		

15 minute chair massages are only $15 or
30 minutes for only $30!

Ask [your contact's name] for more details.

Depending on how much interest and how many chair massages you can effectively administer, you can set up your scheduled times for however long you like (9:40–5:20). Also, notice that I schedule the 15-minute appointments in 20-minute intervals. This gives you some time to breathe between massages, and your clients can get from their desks to you with a minute or two to spare. You don't want to schedule clients in 15-minute intervals, because you will surely get backed up with the first two people and you will get clients waiting for you outside your door. This is not a good situation. People don't like to have their time wasted, waiting for a chair massage and it stresses them out. You should be rested and ready for each person. If you feel rushed, your clients won't like the feeling of you racing through their massage just trying to catch up all day.

2. While setting up your chair, talk to your contact person about benefits, and answer any questions or concerns they might have.

3. Give chair massage. Fifteen minutes should be fine. That's what you are selling, so remember to know your massage routine. I like to bring some recorded new-age music to create that "relaxed" state of mind for the massage.

4. After chair massage, suggest that your contact send out an email to find out who might be interested in chair massage. They might just want to set up a date right away - that's the best situation. Suggest dates and times in the next

two weeks that will be convenient for them and you to return. Leave sign-up sheets with times established (11:00–3:00, let's say). Ask to be set up in a clean, quiet, and private office or conference room. If none are available, make do with wherever they can put you! I have massaged everywhere from rooftops to utility closets. I'm just happy to be on the premises!

If they agree to send out an email, hopefully you will get a good few people interested. But when you call to find out what the response was, don't be discouraged if only two or three people responded. You still should go to work on those few people who are interested, because after the first time you come in, they will have already spread the word about how great your massage was. Then you will be busier every time you return just by word of mouth.

5. Follow up with a phone call or email to your contact person the day before you are scheduled to go in.

Who do you know?

Friends, family, people at the gym, former coworkers, people that are on your softball team. Anyone who has a job at a business is a potential client.

"Back Door" Method

Explain to a friend or acquaintance that you're trying to expand your chair-massage practice and that you would like to give her a free massage at work. Ask your friend to check with the supervisor/manager to make sure it's okay.

Mention that your friend could say that you "owe" a massage for a favor that she did for you. Show up at the prearranged time and give the massage. After the massage, make sure your friend introduces you to the supervisor, and thank her for letting you in the door. Just in case, have cards and brochures handy to give out and thank her again.

Wait a day or two, and then send the supervisor your cover letter, resume, business cards, and brochure with all the pertinent information. Say in the letter that you would love to give her a complimentary massage to see how wonderful it is. This person has seen your face, knows what you do, and has already met you. That's a lot of good things going for you!

Get that person on the phone and get that meeting. Maybe, she will just book you!

Other Venues – different approaches

Flea Markets, Retail Stores, Health Food Stores etc.

If you have good people skills, finding work with a **retail store** is all about confidence and presentation. But basically:

Ask to see the manager. If it is a flea market or farmer's market, you should ask one of the vendors about getting your own booth. Introduce yourself and present your business card and services.

Tell them you would be interested in setting up in a small area and offering chair massage to the customers who are willing to pay for it. Let's say you keep 70 percent and give the rest to the business. It's up to you to negotiate what you are willing to share with the business. If you feel lucky, maybe start out by offering 10 percent to the business. Or you might even say that it would give the store a "healthy" reputation (which it will) that will be good for their business. Offering discounts to employees will also make your services more attractive.

As long as you are an independent contractor, you will handle any money transactions and settle up by the end of each shift.

Have a sign-up sheet where you keep track of your client's name and minutes spent with you. Try handing out small flyers that give away "FREE 2 minutes of chair massage from 1:20–1:50 today!" This will attract people to your chair for their free two minutes, but most people will want more time. Always ask at the end of the two minutes, "Would you like a quick five more minutes? It's only a dollar a minute!"

Show up at your designated time and location in the store, and bring a sign that says, "Chair Massage $1 a minute, by Mark Worrell, CMT. No appointment necessary."

Be there on time consistently for every shift whether it's once a week or five days a week. Ask if you can use the PA system to make announcements about your presence. Offer those "free two minutes **right now**" over the PA system and you will usually get someone sitting down right away.

Back in 1996, I started doing chair massage two days a week at a healthy grocery-food store. The shift was from 3:00 p.m. to 7:00 p.m. During the first few months, making announcements, handing out flyers for "Free 2 Minutes," I was pulling in only $40 per day. But because I was consistent and people could count on me being there, by the time I left in 2001, I was averaging about $150 a shift and had landed three chair-massage accounts out of it.

If you're looking into setting up in a shopping mall, you need to check with the mall's sales manager to discuss overhead: cost of renting a space (kiosk), insurance information, and time involved in the lease agreement. Obviously, they have set mall hours when you must be present. Find out if you need to hire other therapists to cover any shifts. Calculate the costs of buying the massage chairs, massage insurance, supplies, and advertising costs. You'll have to work out how much you need to make each day, each week, and each month to stay afloat.

Conventions, Trade Shows, etc.

If you live in a big city or area with venues for conventions and trade shows, the following is a simple way of finding out about upcoming conventions. Call the venue; let's say the Kansas City convention center. Ask to speak with the director of operations and see if he or she handles all upcoming events. Explain who you are and that you are interested in setting up a booth for chair massage. Be prepared to answer any questions about costs so have a quote ready. You and that person must then decide if you will charge the attendees directly or if the venue will pick up the cost.

Another angle is to offer to be present in the convention as a complimentary service. But, you will have to refer to the "Fish Bowl" section below to gather contacts for giving a free chair massage. You have to decide if it is worth your effort to give free massages. If the convention is national, it might not be worth your time if your potential clients live in another part of the state or out of state. You should offer complimentary chair massages only if you can expect some future business out of it. You want to ask about local conventions or exhibits that deal with businesses in your geographical area.

Get the information I have introduced earlier in this book from whomever you speak with. Follow up with that person and maybe offer a free chair massage so he or she can meet you. Heck, you might get a massage account at the venue's corporate offices.

"Fish Bowl" of Business

Hopefully, with what I have already talked about in getting a chair-massage business going into a flea market or retail establishment, this next part is easy!

Say you are doing chair massage at a health food grocery store. On your table on which you have set up your information, sign with title and massage price, and sign-up sheet, place a fish bowl with another small sign that says, "WIN a free chair massage in your office! Place business card in here!"

People then put their business cards in the fish bowl. You see where I am getting to, don't you? Take these business cards once, twice, or three times a week and pick a name. Call that person and tell her that she has WON! All she has to do is get permission from her supervisor for you to come in with your chair in the next day or two. Set up a time and go in to give the free chair massage. You can do this as many times as you like in a week. It keeps you busy and people get to know who you are.

After the massage, do what you have done in "Back Door Method" and ask to see the supervisor. Thank her and go on your merry way. Send in your information ASAP and try to get that meeting!

Another way of getting in the door is to mail your massage packet to every business card you get! Those people know that you're the massage guy at the health food store because you will state that in the cover letter. Let them know that you would love it if they could forward your packet to their human resources or office managers. If they oblige, even though they didn't "win" this month's free office massage, you would still like to come in to give them a free massage anyway. Remember, you want to get into the business. That is the most effective way to get that account.

Websites and Social Networking

This part of the book is one that has been talked about and analyzed by myself, students, and working therapists.

First, you can let all of your friends know on let's say, Facebook, what you are doing by setting up a personal page with all your information. Having all your friends let their friends know that you're starting to go to workplaces to do chair massage and that you would really appreciate any referrals. This is pretty obvious to get your friends to help you, but don't expect everyone to jump onboard right away. However, you can say "hello" on Facebook every few days to different friends, specifically mentioning to them that you would love to come by their office to give them a chair massage. Free massages are always appreciated and you might get an account this way.

Go through the Facebook ad platform. Part of the Facebook ad platform lets you target your advertising. You don't actually have to launch an ad in order to take advantage of this feature. Part of the process for setting up a Facebook ad allows you to target your ad to specific demographics or audiences based on their interests, age, gender, or location— all sorts of different factors. Part of that targeting actually gives you a number of the people who fit those criteria. So it's definitely a great, free way to find out a ballpark number for who fits your target market.

Having your website and buying ads on Google is very easy to do. They have step-by-step directions on how to set up and geo-locate for your area, but you will be paying "per click," which can be very expensive. So, have a good idea of how much you want to spend on ads every day and set a budget!

I want to share with you the best ways of marketing chair massage online, but I want to point out my feelings on web-*only* marketing. In the previous pages, doing the work and sending out packages to your target is going out and "getting" business. Websites require people trying to search you out. But remember, we are not a service that is widely known about. If they are not looking for your services, they are not going to search online. You need to notify them of your existence. It's still a unique service that people need to learn about having at their workplace.

In the last few years, having your own website and keeping up your Facebook friendships is all good and well. But to tell you the truth, trying to promote a massage business using only websites doesn't really work. I have done the research by talking with other therapists who have tried to market themselves online only, and have found that they have created NO NEW BUSINESS accounts. Using online marketing in addition to your massage packages can be useful though.

Massage therapy is such a "personal" service, people don't hire you based on how professional your website looks. They need to meet you in person to really get who you are. If you have a website that describes you and your services, you can add that in your business letter and brochure. But just having a website and blogging on Facebook or advertising on Google is not cost-effective. Those "pay per click" ads can add up very quickly if this is the only way you market yourself. The other problem with trying to get chair-massage accounts through online methods only is that you can't go just anywhere your potential clients are. Geographically, you want to get accounts that you are in close proximity with. Let's say someone clicks on your website and actually decides to contact you. But her business is 70 miles away from you. Even using the ads online to target just your city may not let you distinguish how far you are from potential clients (in miles). It would be hardly worth your time and gas money to travel that far, when there are businesses you can approach in your area with massage packages. Advertising online only for business within 25 miles of you is impossible to target when someone can just click on your website, costing you 25 cents per click. Forget the cost of keeping your website running. For the time, effort, and money, therapists I know who have tried regret the investment.

Part Three:
Maintaining your Accounts

On Massage Day

1. Show up half an hour early. You want get there and have enough time to set up the chair. Time to get a copy of the sign-up sheet. Time to get a glass of water or refreshment. Time to use the restroom, if needed.

2. Make sure to bring your lotion, music, and hand disinfectant. Depending on your training, some therapists use a light moisturizing lotion to work on the arms and hands. A CD or MP3 player and some speakers playing soothing new-age music add a nice element to let your clients "float away." You want to show each client that you are thinking about cleanliness and basic hygiene by using a simple disinfectant gel in between massages.

3. Greet clients and ask, *"Have you ever had a chair massage before?"* Most of the time they will answer that they haven't. I like to say something like, *"It's easy! You get to sit here and I do all the work!"* Besides a nice massage, you want to be there to make people feel at ease. Another thing I like to say is, *"Just sit down and I'll take care of you."*

4. If necessary, show them how to sit on the massage chair. A lot of people who are new to massage don't know how to sit in a contraption like a massage

chair. Don't let them be embarrassed by sitting on it backwards! Quickly show them how to sit and lean into the face cradle.

5. Do your massage. Check in with them about the pressure! So many therapists have this idea that, *"I was trained professionally and I know what my clients want!"* You don't know who is sensitive to deep pressure or likes deeper work. You don't know if some people have a bruise under their shirts or if they had a heavy workout that day and are really sore. Ask them at least twice, *"How's that pressure?"* or *"Is that pressure okay?"* Don't let your ego get in the way of opening up that good line of communication with a new client.

6. After the massage, thank them and let them know when you will be back. If you're not sure of your next date, mention to them that you hope to be back in the next two weeks to a month. You'll want to also encourage them to speak to your contact person and mention how much they enjoyed the visit. And don't be afraid to have your new clients mention it to their coworkers. Learn this phrase: *"I hope that you enjoyed your massage and mention your experience to your coworkers."* Just reading it sounds silly, but when you say it out loud, it makes for perfectly good "breezy" conversation.

7. **VERY IMPORTANT**: Try not to "push" any products or even your full-body massages on your clients. You will surely deter any future visits if you try to sell them on something they never asked for. Only hand out your business cards when asked. Don't give any diagnosis for any ailments they

might have. You are not a licensed doctor and could be held liable if you recommend any medications that might have an adverse affect on your client. This includes recommending any herbal substitutes.

In-Office Promotional Flyer/Email

After you have started out at a new account, hopefully, you have been promoted by your contact person through emails that let the company know your scheduled dates and times. But after a while, things might level out a bit. To boost your account and promote from within, see about sending your contact person a "sales" email. In this email you'll want address the issue of stress at work and how massage is the answer. People need to know your name and what your services are all about. They need to know how often you visit. They need to know your rates, or if the company is doing shared or full cost.

If email is not the way to go, you should check with your contact person and see if you can post a paper flyer (printed on blue or yellow paper for maximum attention) in the company's lunch rooms and satellite areas. You might even ask if you can drop off a flyer in everyone's "in" box. Just make sure it's ok for you to walk into every area of the workplace. You don't want to walk into a conference room where an important meeting might be taking place. My in-house flyers/emails look like this:

☺ ☺ ☺ ☺ ☺ ☺

[Company name] employees!

Give yourself a deserved stress break!

You can get a professional
massage right here at work!

Relax and rejuvenate yourself!
It's much healthier than any
coffee or cigarette break.
Every two weeks or so, **Mark Worrell,
C.MT.,** is available for chair massage.
Get a wonderful back, neck, arms,
and hands chair massage next Thursday.
Appointments from 11:00–3:00.
Sessions are only **$15 for 15 minutes
Or $30 for 30 minutes**.

(your contact's name and ext. #) has more details.
Look out for emails about dates and times!

☺ ☺ ☺ ☺ ☺ ☺

Pricing

Best advice: Start out low. Go for "volume" to work on more people sooner, rather than the "quick buck." When you first start out in any business, your "edge" might just be that you are so reasonably priced, people can't refuse or claim finances as an excuse NOT to get worked on.

The average going rate for chair massage is about a dollar a minute, depending on if you're in a "big city" or rural area. But offering it at $12 for 15 minutes will surely get more people in your chair quicker than expecting them to pay $20 when they have never met you or have never had a professional massage therapist work on them.

If you feel, in the next six months, that you have enough "regulars," you can surely raise your price by a dollar or two. Don't expect to keep everybody as a client. Finances may be an issue. I suggest that you email or call each individual client when you plan to raise the rate.

Setting Goals

How many chair massages per day do you want to give? How many clients do you want to see in a week? How many different accounts do you want in the next six months? Break up your goals into daily, weekly, monthly, and yearly. Keeping track of your chair massages gives you something to shoot for every week. Last week you did 12 chair massages, so this week you have to go for 15. Yesterday you made $75, so today you'll go for $90. Having these goals will push you into acquiring more accounts, making more phone calls, and help keep you busy.

Networking

Keep in contact with as many therapists as possible. Get together with leads on new spas that might be opening or new businesses in the area that might be able to use your services. Discuss your goals openly with your therapist colleagues and follow up on your goals and theirs. Throw out any and all ideas on making your business prosper. Many therapists who might be busy for a day will eventually refer you out to handle any overload.

The more therapists you keep in contact with, the more you will expand your chances of any new leads. Helping out someone else not only is the right way of doing business, but it will also return to you with business opportunities of your own.

At social occasions, always have business cards available. You never know who might work at a large corporation and is looking for something new to offer to employees.

You can also join up with your local networking clubs. You can search them on the Internet or in local papers. A networking group is a group of business owners that gets together for weekly meetings discussing their businesses with each other. The idea is that they will refer you to people, and you do the like for them. There usually is a small fee to join a club, or you just pay for your own breakfast wherever you might meet up. It could be a small group of five to six people or as big as 40–50 people out of whom you might be able to get business. You don't want to join a group if they already have a massage practitioner because that would be a "conflict of interest." They usually prescreen you to find out what kind of business you do anyway.

Check out the following online:

Business Network International   www.bni.com
LEADS   www.leads.com
LeTip International   www.letip.com

If you decide to join a networking group, make sure you are consistent with attending meetings. Always have business cards or brochures handy. Show up early for meetings and introduce yourself to everybody. Follow up with contacts you make, even if it is just to say, *"Hi John, it was nice meeting you yesterday at the BNI group!"* Plan to refer the people you met and their businesses. If people do refer you, make sure to follow up with a thank-you email or call. They will appreciate it and you will look gracious. Maybe offer them a free chair or full-body massage when they refer you. That's bound to get some good return.

Promoting Full Body

Well, now comes the easy part. You've got yourself an account. They already know your outstanding work. They're comfortable with you. You've proven yourself dependable. People will probably ask for your business card anyway. This is a no-brainer. Once people get a sample, they usually want more.

Have your full-body rate comparable to your chair rates. Don't quote different people different rates as they might trade notes about you. You don't want to have to explain why "client A" has to pay $65 for an hour when "client B" is only paying $50.

If you're available for privates, at their home or yours, discuss your availability. If you work at a spa that you want to have them visit, give them that information. Let's say that you have a personal problem with a chair client and you don't really want to work on this person privately. What do you say? Well, the best way is to let her know that you are not taking any private clients at this time, and that you would love to refer her to another therapist in the area.

Now is the right time

I have personally tried all of these marketing strategies for finding corporate accounts. Obviously, I have only included the ones that work the best. The only way you'll find out if they work is by doing it. My hope is that you will find new business and prosper.

I wish you all the luck and good fortune in your quest to start your own chair-massage business. I hope that, the more massage gets out there, the more businesses will accept massage as an efficient and cost-effective way to take care of their employees.

Technique

In the past 16 years I have performed over 18,000 "documented" 15-minute chair massages. That is to say that I have kept all my sign-up sheets filed away and have counted each one. I can tell you on any given work day how many clients I worked on, where I worked, and how much money I made that day. I'm not sure why I first started saving the sheets, but I think it was for my own interest in my numbers for any given year. My biggest year was 2007 where I worked on 1,492 clients. Mind you, those are not 1,492 different people—they are all repeat clients at a little over 12 accounts throughout the year. I think that my endurance and stamina was built up over the years because of my "hand-saving" techniques, which I am sharing with you here and on **Youtube.com** for free. Search for "**Chair Massage Everywhere – Technique and Marketing book**" to check it out. The great thing with the Youtube video is you can play it as many times as you need to get a good idea of my technique and can develop your own routine based on these highlights.

I have given the strokes different, creative, maybe even silly names for the sake of memory. They work as "anchors" so I you can easily remember them if called upon to do so. Anyway, how boring is it to say "open hand thumb knead" when I can give it a name like "ten pipers piping?" All of these techniques have been learned from other therapists I have worked with through the years and my own experimentation. I have always recommended to my students that they should practice a routine at least 25–30 times before feeling confident to get out and charge people.

They might not make much sense here just reading them, but in conjunction with the Youtube video, hopefully it all makes sense.

"Cat Crawl"

Application area: Top of shoulders-trapezius
Therapist position: Head of massage chair

Kneading/compressions with heels of hands and thumbs. "Swaying" with your own body weight for pressure.

"C" Hands

Appl. Area: Top of neck, base of skull
Ther. Pos.:   Head of massage chair

Hands/fingers in the letter "c" position, stay firm, small circles, frictions to the occipital ridge, leaning back to use your own body weight for pressure.

Flat Fists

Appl. Area: Start at top of back, down to sacrum
Ther. Pos.:   Back of massage chair

With arms extended in locked position, hands are flat fists on either side of spine. Compressions down back to top of sacrum. Thumbs are positioned on the erectors.

"Ten Pipers Piping"

Appl. Area: Mid thoracic area, up to top of shoulders
Ther. Pos.:   Back of chair starting with left side of client's body

Open hand thumb knead, left hand above right (right hand above left when you work on to the right side), thumbs are 1 to 2 inches apart, starting mid-thoracic, left side of spine on erectors working your way up to top of shoulders, then round back to where you started. Arms are straight out, locked position, "swaying" with your own weight for pressure.

Heel palm press

Appl. Area.:   Mid thoracic area, up to top of shoulder
Ther. Pos.:   Back of chair, left side, arms locked

Using heel of the hand, compressions to left side of spine, up to top of shoulder.

Transition into:

4 points and 4 "rollovers" – Upper back

Appl. Area: Mid thoracic area, to top of shoulders
Ther. Pos.:   Left side of chair, nice open stance into position. Keep your back straight.

Using your tip of right elbow and forearm, step up with open stance, sink into left side of spine, small circles away from erectors, moving up to hit 4 points to the top of shoulder.

Top of shoulder, tip of elbow, rolling over trapezius 4 times. You're going for that "golf ball" knot that pretty much everyone has on the top of the shoulder.

Transition over to right side of client's body, right side of chair with "Ten Pipers Piping."

Apply, **ten pipers piping, heel palm press, 4 points** and **4 rollovers** to right side of client's body using left elbow for 4 points and 4 rollovers.

You will do this transitioning back and forth from left side to right side in this combination of strokes, about 3–4 times in a 15-minute routine. After third or fourth time, ending on the right side, transition into:

4 points top of neck

Appl. Area: Top of neck, base of skull
Ther. Pos.:   Right side of chair, left hand

Using your left hand, hit 4 points on occipital ridge with thumb, starting from distally to medially – twice. Then, knead down the neck in 4 points – twice.

Transition from right side of chair, using right hand applied to neck, to circle around back of chair to left side.

Right hand, hit 4 points on occipital ridge with thumb, starting distally to medially – twice. Then, knead down the neck in 4 points – twice.

Without losing contact with client's neck, circle around to head of massage chair. Transition into:

"C" Hands

Transition into:

Scalp knead

Appl. Area: Head, scalp
Ther. Pos.:   Head of massage chair, both hands

Simple kneading with fingers, moving hands in circular motions in 3–4 different areas on head.

Transition into:

"Cat Crawl"

Without losing contact, circle around to left side of chair, getting ready to work on left arm of client. Transition into:

"Duck Bills"

Appl. Area: Left upper arm
Ther. Pos.:   Left side of chair, both hands

Kneading deltoid, biceps, and triceps at same time down and back up arm, 3–4 times. Fingers on the underside, thumbs on the outsides. Thumbs should be pointing down toward floor.

As you take a seat, don't lose contact. Transition into:

4 points on forearm, milking forearm

Appl. Area: Left forearm
Ther. Pos.:   Sitting in chair, thumbs on the
                        outside of forearm, fingers on the
                        inside

Apply compressions with hands, thumbs on top of client's forearms and fingers wrapped around forearm on inside. Compress (squeeze) in 4 points – twice.

Left hand rests on client's left hand, while you reach for moisture lotion and apply to your own hand. Milk forearm by holding client's left wrist with your left hand and milking left forearm with right hand, with concentration of pressure with your thumb 3–4 times.

Spreading of hands and wringing of fingers

Appl. Area: Client's left hand
Ther. Pos.:   Still sitting, using both hands

Spread out client's hand with your hands, with your heel of hands, fingers wrapping around client's hand, kneading, pulling, spreading out palms.

With your right hand, wrap around client's pinky finger and pull slowly down to tip. Continue to next 2 fingers, then switching to your left hand to get index finger and thumb.

With left hand, hit 4 points on forearm, while standing up, right hand goes to top of back, standing up to circle around back of chair, smoothing out shoulders as you transition to right side of chair working on client's right upper arm:

"Duck Bills"

Transition into:

4 points on forearm, milking forearm

This time, lotion your own hand, milk forearm by holding client's right wrist, with your right hand and milking with your left hand, with concentration of pressure with your thumb 3–4 times.

Transition into:

Spreading of hands, wringing of fingers

This time, with your left hand, wrap around client's pinky finger and pull slowly down to tip. Continue to next 2 fingers, then switching to your right hand to do index finger and thumb.

With right hand, hit 4 points on forearm, while standing up, left hand goes to top of back, standing up to circle around back of chair, smoothing out shoulders as you transition to center back of chair:

Flat Fists down to sacrum twice.

Pull out kneeling pad from underneath chair, take a knee, transition into:

4 points lower back

Appl. Area: Mid thoracic to sacrum
Ther. Pos.:   Kneeling, right elbow

Tip of right elbow starting mid-thoracic, left side of client's spine, hit 4 points working away from erectors, down to top of sacrum. Use "sway" with your own weight for pressure. Repeat 4 points, 4 times.

Flat fists to lower back

Appl. Area: Mid-thoracic to top of sacrum
Ther. Pos.:   Kneeling, flat fists with hands

While still kneeling, apply flat fists to lower back, with arms bent, making small circles away from spine, with hands on either side of spine, in 4 points. Repeat 4 times.

"Butterfly" hands

Appl. Area: Mid-thoracic to sacrum
Ther. Pos.:   Kneeling, hands spread out with
                                  butterfly shape

Still kneeling, hands start either side mid-thoracic to sacrum, 4 points, 4 times.

"Swimming Turtles"

Appl. Area: Mid-thoracic to sacrum
Ther. Pos.:   Kneeling, hands form turtle-shell shape

Kneeling, hands form a turtle-shell shape, starting mid-thoracic. Pressure point comes from corner of palms of hands, close to pisiform bone. Pulling away from spine in circular motion, 4 points down to sacrum. Repeat 4 times.

Smooth out area with flat hands, while standing. Transition into:

Left side **ten pipers piping, heel palm press, 4 points, and 4 rollovers** over to right side **ten pipers piping, heel palm press, 4 points, and 4 rollovers.** Repeat this combination at least 2 times.

Transition into right side of chair into:

4 points top of neck

Circle around backside of chair into:

4 points top of neck with right hand.

Transition into:

"C" hands

Scalp knead into:

Cat Crawl

51

Then, come to left side of chair into:

Balancing

Appl. Area: Entire back
Ther. Pos.:   Left hand top of back, right hand on sacrum

Standing on left side of chair, left hand is at the top of the back, right hand on sacrum. Rocking client in chair back and forth.

Come around to back of chair, smooth out upper back, squeezing deltoids.

Immediately start:

Percussions

Appl. Area: Entire back
Ther. Pos.:   Standing at back of chair,
                         pummeling and hacking

Pummeling: Hands are loose fists, with thumbs up, heavy taps to client's back, down and back up.

Hacking: Hands are in flat position, palms against each other, with loose fingers, heavy taps to client's back.

Smooth out shoulders, then light, rapid strokes down the back, 7–8 times (ask your client to "take a nice, deep breath"), and then one, rapid light stroke down arms.

You've done it!

I know this might seem really confusing, but if you watch the video, you can learn that much quicker. Again, that's "**Chair Massage Everywhere – Technique and Marketing Book**" and doing it over and over. Maybe have someone sit in your massage chair to practice on and another person to read, line by line, from this book.

Try to practice all of these techniques, one by one. Work on the transitions to the next stroke after you feel confident with each separate stroke.

Now, good luck and go get 'em so we have Chair Massage Everywhere! Best wishes to you all!

www.ingramcontent.com/pod-product-compliance
Lightning Source LLC
Chambersburg PA
CBHW020331290526
45785CB00007B/3003